Homemade Deodorants and Body Sprays

35 Refreshing Non-Toxic Recipes

Table of Contents

Introduction

I would like to thank and congratulate you for downloading *"DIY Deodorants: 35 Refreshing, Non-Toxic, Homemade, Deo and Body Spray Recipes to Help You Stay Fresh 24/7.* I can honestly say that you have taken a positive step towards making healthier choices in the products you use to smell better and thus feel better.

You are going to feel so much better and safer using your own non-toxic homemade deodorants and body sprays I cannot begin to tell you. Not to mention saving a big chunk of change on what you would normally spend on commercial products of this nature.

Feel good in knowing that the recipes in this book are safe and do not come with a risk of developing liver disease, or breast cancer as well as many other terrible health complications!

No worries here you can feel safe in knowing that the recipes in this book are not going to cause you any harm or increase your chances of developing some kind of cancer or other awful ailment. Instead enjoy these recipes within these pages, even add some extra ingredients to them to make them your own—have fun with it!

Chapter 1. Why You Should Use Organic Ingredients

Applying deodorant is for many of us just another part of our daily ritual, it is something most of us do not put too much thought into. It comes in different forms such as roll on stick or liquid roll on, or a spray.

It is mainly used to prevent the awful offensive smell of sweaty body odor. It helps make sure that when you lift your arm up there is not going to be an awful smell drifting into the face of a nearby by stander. Deodorant helps to defend against you developing wet underarms and stinky armpits. This is all well in good, the problem lies in the ingredients of the deodorant products we are using.

We are going to have a look at some of the conventional deodorant ingredients, and then you will decide if these sweat blocking additives are what you really want spread across your bare skin all day. Once you have a better understanding of the ingredients in conventional deodorants I think you will be much more inclined to want to make your own non-toxic deodorants.

Aluminum

The main ingredient used in antiperspirant deodorants is *aluminum*. This metal is used to block your sweat glands, this metal causes you to decrease your sweat capability by about twenty percent. The serious problems connected to this metal is that is can end up causing serious health risks such as Alzheimer's disease and breast cancer.

So you must be wondering 'if the aluminium is blocking my sweat what happens to it?' Our under arms are closely linked to lymph nodes, so this accumulation of toxins from your sweat no being perspired as it should can have the potential to cause major problems in your armpits.

When there is a build-up of toxins in your body this in turn can cause cell mutation.

There is controversial studies about the links to aluminium and breast cancer. With this being said the most common areas of breast cancer develop in the upper outer quadrants of the breasts, which is close to the armpits where the lymph nodes are located.

It seems to show that long-term use of deodorants with aluminium are linked to the formation of certain breast cancers. Also making it easier for the aluminium to pass through the under arm area is the fact that many women shave their underarms.

Phthalates

This is an ingredient that is used as a fragrance, it is a plasticizing chemical that is used in many beauty products due to its ability to help dissolve some of the other ingredients in the products. This product will help the deodorant to glide on nice and smoothly. This smooth glide comes with links that could lead to larger problems later on.

Phthalates have been linked to many health issues and they are considered to be endocrine disruptors. Once your body has absorbed them they act much like estrogen, which not only conflict with normal hormonal function, but they can also lead to many other complications such as:

- Infertility
- Allergies
- Endometriosis
- Asthma
- Lung, kidney and liver damage
- Prostrate, ovarian, and breast cancer
- Decreased sperm count

These commercial deodorant products are probable human carcinogens they are going to continue to be sold while the United States continues to regulate them, being ingredients in many beauty products, including deodorants. I am sure you are like most people and did not even take into consideration that the products that you have been using on your skin for years might indeed be a risk to your health.

Products such as deodorants are just another one of those endless pitfalls in the endless array of chemicals that are having a negative effect on our health and they continue to be added into many conventional skin care products.

Now is the time for you to put these commercial products aside that are risking your health and in their place choose to make some non-toxic deodorants and body sprays by following the recipes that I have collected for your use within these pages.

Feel good in knowing that these homemade products are not going to possibly cause any kind of cancer or other serious ailment to you or your loved ones! Now let us move on to the next chapter and take a look at this wonderful collection of non-toxic, homemade, organic deodorants and body sprays

!

Chapter 2. Collection of Organic Deodorant Recipes

1. Shea Butter Deodorant

Ingredients:

- two tablespoons of Arrowroot powder

- three tablespoons of baking soda

- two tablespoons of Shea butter

- three tablespoons of coconut oil

- Essential oil of your choice

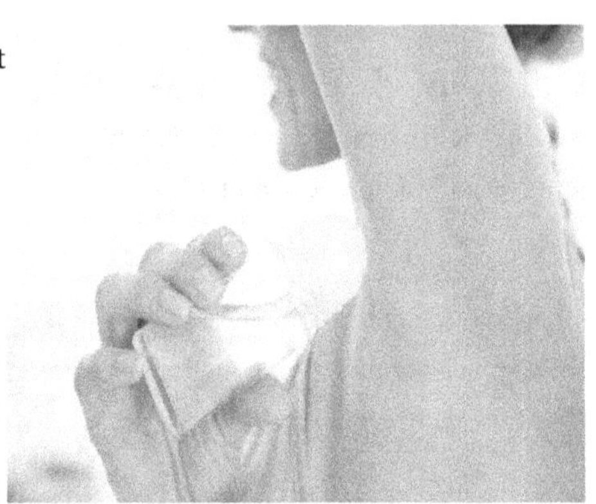

Directions:

In a double broiler over medium heat melt your Shea butter and coconut oil. Combine them in a mason jar placing into the broiler. Remove from heat and add in your arrowroot and baking soda.

Mix well. Add in your choice of essential oils. Pour into a glass container to store. You do not have to refrigerate. You may choose to put it into an old deodorant stick once it has cooled completely for easier use. You can speed up the hardening process by putting it into the fridge.

2. *Vitamin E Deodorant*

Ingredients:

- two tablespoons of cornstarch

- three tablespoons of Shea butter

- three tablespoons of baking soda

- two vitamin E caps

- two tablespoons of cocoa butter

- essential oil of your choice, about 15-20 drops

Directions:

Melt all of your ingredients except for the essential oil, and mix well. Remove from heat and add in the essential oil, mix well. Put into glass jar and allow to set in the refrigerator.

3. *Simple Deodorant*

Ingredients:

- one quarter cup of arrowroot powder

- five tablespoon of coconut oil

- one quarter cup of baking soda

Directions:

Mix arrowroot powder and baking soda then add in coconut oil mixing it into a paste. You can store in a small container or put into an empty deodorant stick for use.

4. ***DIY Natural Solid Deodorant***

Ingredients:

- one tablespoon of beeswax

- two tablespoons of coconut oil

- one tablespoon of Shea butter

- three drops of Citronella essential oil

- three drops of lemongrass essential oil

- one tablespoon of baking soda

- one and a half tablespoons of Bentonite clay

- two tablespoons of arrowroot powder

- three drops of Tea tree essential oil

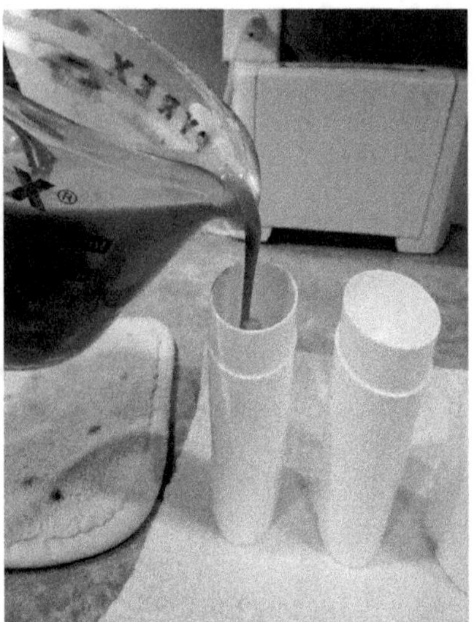

Directions:

In a double broiler add in your bees wax, coconut oil and Shea butter over medium heat, stir until the wax and oils have melted. Remove mix from heat and add in your essential oils, arrowroot powder, Bentonite clay and mix well.

Pour this liquid into some silicone muffin molds or an empty deodorant container and allow to cool down and solidify for about three hours. The bees wax is going to help keep it solid so you can use it like a traditional deodorant.

*5. **Natural Coconut Deodorant***

Ingredients:

- one eighth of a cup of arrowroot powder

- one eighth of a cup of cornstarch

- one quarter of a cup of coconut oil

- one tablespoon of baking soda

- essential oils of your choice, about ten drops

Directions:

In a mixing bowl add cornstarch, coconut oil, baking soda, arrowroot powder and mix well. Add in your essential oils and mix.

Pour mix into an empty deodorant container or into a small mason jar and place in the fridge for twenty minutes. Remove from fridge as use as needed.

*6. **Detoxifying Natural Deodorant***

Ingredients:

- two tablespoons of Bentonite clay

- four tablespoons of arrowroot powder

- four tablespoons of baking soda

- six tablespoons of coconut oil

- 20 drops of Tea tree essential oil

Directions:

Add all of your ingredients into a mixing bowl and blend well. Heat the coconut oil first so that it will mix easily with other ingredients. Knead the mixture with your hands to make it into a smooth paste.

Add to empty deodorant stick or glass jar. Allow it to cool. Scoop out with finger when you want to apply the paste. Rub paste under arms it will melt quickly into your skin.

7. Rubbing Alcohol

Ingredients:

- Rubbing alcohol
- cotton balls
- optional 20 drops of your choice of essential oil

Directions:

You can kill the odor causing bacteria by using this inexpensive way of helping to fight this problem. Just fill a spray bottle with rubbing alcohol then spritz your underarms, or you can choose to dab it on with a cotton ball.

You can also add some of your favorite essential oil to make it smell more pleasing.

8. Lemon Juice Deodorant

Ingredients:

- lemon juice

Directions:

Lemon juice is a great natural deodorizer that many people enjoy making use of. In the lemon juice is citric acid that helps to kill the odor-causing bacteria under your arms. Use a slice of lemon on your armpits in the morning. You may also collect the juice in a spray bottle and spritz the juice on to your underarms. Keep in mind not to use the lemon juice on areas that have recently been shaved.

9. All-Natural Homemade Deodorant

Ingredients:

- one eighth of a cup of arrowroot powder
- one eighth of a cup of cocoa butter
- half a tablespoon of baking soda
- six drops of vitamin E oil
- one eighth of cup of Shea Butter
- 25 drops of your choice of essential oil

Directions:

Combine your cocoa butter and Shea butter, mix well. Use a double broiler to heat oil over medium heat until they have become melted, blend well. Remove them from heat add in your baking soda, arrowroot powder, vitamin E and essential oil and mix well. Pour mix into two ounce tins, place lid gently on the top do not lock lid at this point. This is just to prevent dust from getting into the mixture while it is in the cooling down process. Leave it to cool down overnight.

10. Summertime Deodorant

Ingredients:

- one quarter of cup of baking soda

- one quarter of a cup of cornstarch

- four tablespoons of coconut oil

- one and a half tablespoons of bees wax, grated

- six Tea tree essential oil drops

- six drops of lavender essential oil

Directions:

Melt your oils in a double broiler over medium heat and stir until melted. Remove from heat then add in the rest of your ingredients. Mix well. Add this paste into an empty deodorant container.

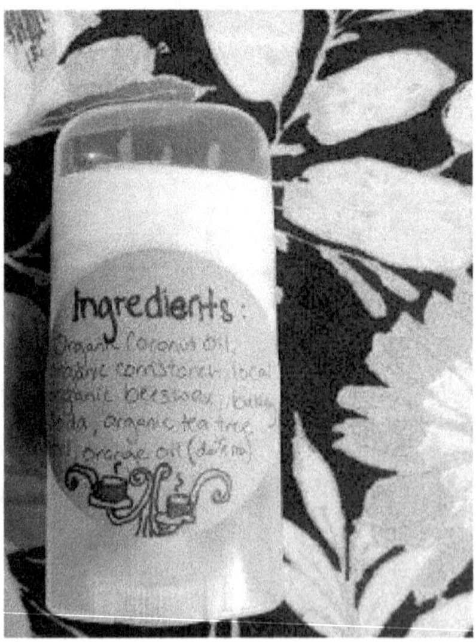

11. Deodorant Bar

Ingredients:

- half a cup of Shea butter

- half a cup of coconut butter

- half a cup of bees wax

- three tablespoons of baking soda

- one and a half teaspoons of vitamin E oil

- three capsules of high quality probiotics

- half a cup of arrowroot powder

- 25 drops of essential oil of your choice

Directions:

In a double broiler add in the Shea butter, coconut oil, and beeswax, over medium heat stir until melted. Remove from heat and add in your arrowroot powder, vitamin E, probiotics, baking soda, and essential oil, mix well. Just make sure before adding these ingredients that the oil is not too hot.

You do not want to kill your probiotics. Gently stir the mix until well blended. Pour into muffin tins or another mold that can hold liquid. If you want to put it into an empty deodorant stick then let it harden in bowl until it turns to be the consistency of peanut butter. Add into empty deodorant stick, scooping and packing it down. Allow cover of stick to stay off overnight to allow it to harden.

12. *Homemade Deodorant*

Ingredients:

- half a cup of baking soda

- half a cup of coconut oil

- 40 drops of your choice of essential oil

- empty deodorant container

Directions:

Put your oil into a bowl and mix baking soda into it. Add in the essential oil and blend well. Fill up the empty deodorant container with mix and leave out overnight with cap off to allow mix to harden.

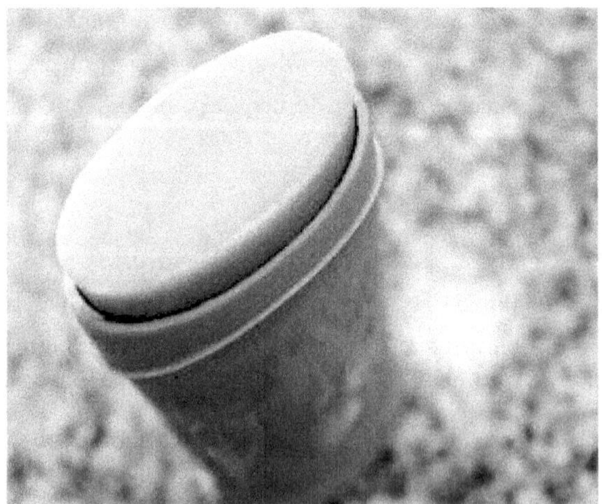

13. Homemade Deodorant for Sensitive Skin

Ingredients:

- one quarter of a cup of Diatomaceous Earth (Food Grade)

- three quarters of a cup of arrowroot powder

- ten tablespoons of melted coconut oil

Directions:

Combine the arrowroot powder with the diatomaceous earth. Mix and keep adding in the melted oil a little at a time. Store in a small glass jar with secure lid use when needed by applying a small amount to your underarms.

14. Sensitive Skin Deodorant

Ingredients:

- seven tablespoons of melted coconut oil

- one quarter of a cup of baking soda

- three quarters of a cup of cornstarch

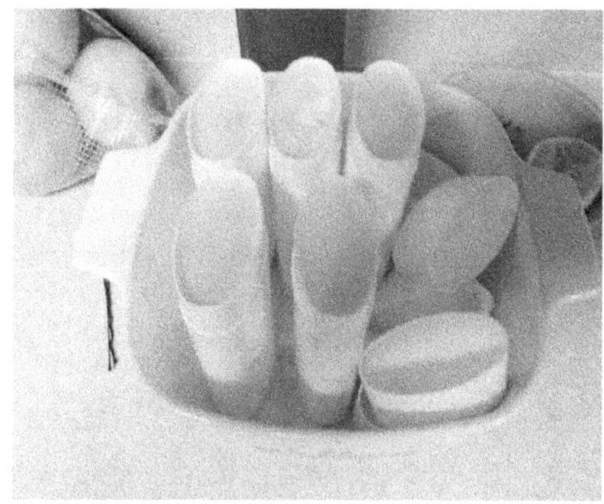

Directions:

Combine your cornstarch with baking soda. Slowly add in the coconut oil a bit at a time blending it in as you go. Use a fork to help mash it down as you progress. Transfer mix to glass jar and seal with secure fitting lid. Apply a little using your fingertips as needed.

15. *Coconut & Lavender Homemade Deodorant*

Ingredients:

- seven tablespoons of coconut oil

- one quarter of a cup of arrowroot powder

- one quarter of a cup of baking soda

- 40 drops of lavender essential oil

Directions:

In a mixing bowl add baking soda, arrowroot powder, mix well, add in coconut oil and lavender essential oil slowly mashing with a fork. You can store the mix in an old deodorant container or in a small glass jar.

16. *Orange Citrus Homemade Deodorant*

Ingredients:

- one and a half teaspoons of bees wax, grated

- four tablespoons of coconut oil

- three tablespoons of Shea butter

- three tablespoons of arrowroot powder

- 35 drops of orange essential oil

Directions:

In a double broiler add in your bees wax, coconut oil and Shea butter, blend until melted. Remove from heat allow to cool down then add in orange essential oil, arrowroot powder and baking soda, blend well. Put mix in empty deodorant container or in small glass jar with secure lid. You can leave over night to allow to harden or you can speed this process up and put it in the fridge for 20 minutes.

17. Grapefruit Homemade Deodorant

Ingredients:

- four tablespoons of Shea butter

- two tablespoons of coconut oil

- one tablespoon of beeswax, grated

- four tablespoons of baking soda

- three tablespoons of arrowroot powder

- 40 drops of grapefruit essential oil

Directions:

In a double broiler add in your Shea butter, coconut oil, and beeswax stir until melted. Remove from heat allowing to cool then add in your baking soda, essential oils, and arrowroot powder mix well.

Add to empty deodorant container for easy use. You can speed up the hardening process by sticking it into the fridge for half an hour. Do not use on areas that have just been shaved.

18. *Grapefruit Body Mist*

Ingredients:

- vodka

- distilled water

- 15 drops of grapefruit essential oil

- dark-glass spray bottle

Directions:

Fill a spray bottle two-thirds with vodka and add in essential oil then top with distilled water and shake before you use.

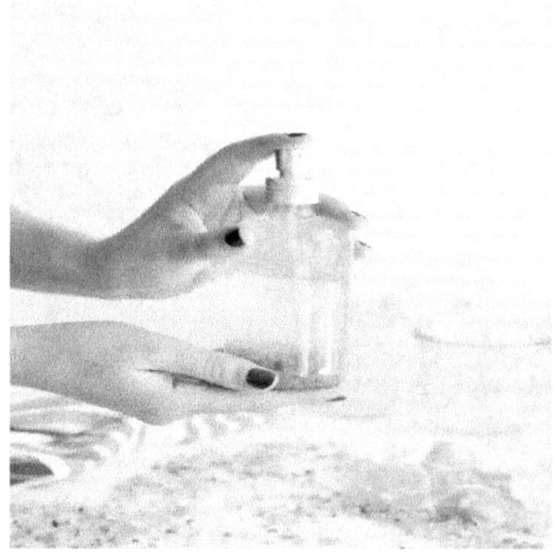

19. *Cardamom & Vanilla Mist*

Ingredients:

- half a cup of distilled water

- one teaspoon of vanilla extract

- six cardamom seeds

Directions:

Crack the cardamom seeds to reveal their pods. Add bits of cardamom to a saucepan with water and bring to a boil.

Remove this from heat. Allow the cardamom water to cool completely. Add scented water to a spray bottle. Add in the vanilla then shake well before using. Store bottle in a cool and dry place.

20. *Tropical Homemade Body Mist*

Ingredients:

- six teaspoons of grapefruit essential oil drops

- 20 Neroli essential oil drops

- one and a half tablespoons of coconut oil

- one and a half tablespoons of vegetable glycerin

- one and a half teaspoons of vodka

- two teaspoons of vanilla extract

- 10ml of Rose Hydrosol

- one and a half ounces of distilled water

Directions:

Fill up a spray bottle with Rose Hydrosol and water. Add in the vegetable glycerin, add in the coconut oil. Mix well. Add in the essential oils close and shake well. Let is rest for a few hours then shake it again before use.

21. *Aloe & Cucumber Body Mist*

Ingredients:

- one cucumber

- one and a half teaspoons of Aloe Vera Gel

- juice from one lemon

- one tablespoon of Rosewater

- distilled water

Directions:

Peel the cucumber and dice it up into little pieces. Place into blender and pulse on high for a minute or so. Cover the bowl with some cheesecloth and then strain the cucumber juice into the bowl.

Add juice to spray bottle. Add the rest of the ingredients and shake well. Store mix in the fridge so it doesn't spoil. It will last about one week.

22. *Forest Scent Body Mist*

Ingredients:

- three drops of fir needle essential oil

- three drops of cedarwood essential oil

- five drops of spruce essential oil

- five drops of Bergamot essential oil

- five drops of Vetiver essential oil

- one teaspoon of Jojoba oil

- distilled water

Directions:

In a spray bottle add in your jojoba oil and essential oils along with some distilled water. Shake well before using.

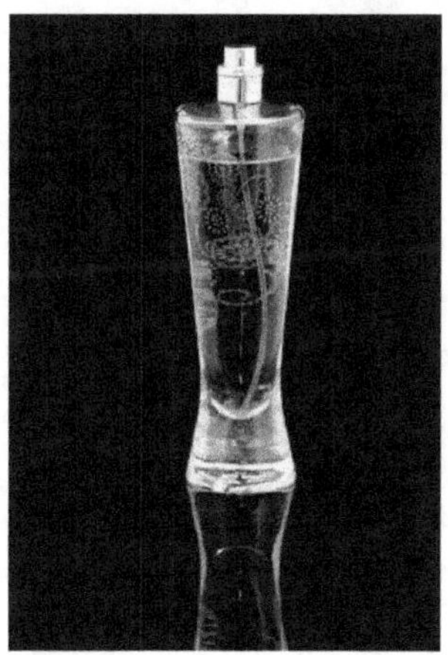

23. *Vanilla, Lemon & Lavender Body Spray*

Ingredients:

- three and a half ounces of witch hazel

- six drops of lemon essential oil

- 35 drops of vanilla essential oil

- 20 drops of Lavender essential oil

Directions:

Add all of your ingredients into a glass spray bottle. Make sure to shake well before every use.

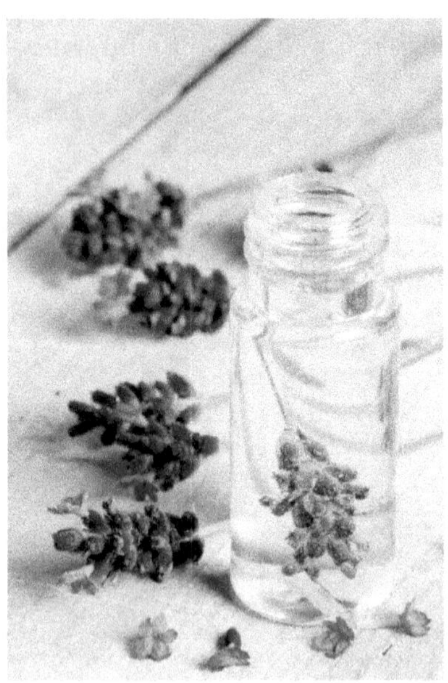

24. *Moisturizing Body Mist*

Ingredients:

- one and a half teaspoons of grapeseed oil

- six drops of vitamin E oil

- two teaspoons of vegetable glycerin

- 20 drops of vanilla essential oil

- one tablespoon of witch hazel

- distilled water

Directions:

Add all of your ingredients into a glass spray bottle and shake well before each use. Great to use just after a shower, rub it into your skin.

25. *Purifying Body Mist*

Ingredients:

- 40 drops of eucalyptus essential oil

- 35 drops of lemon essential oil

- 25 drops of peppermint essential oil

- distilled water

- two tablespoons of witch hazel

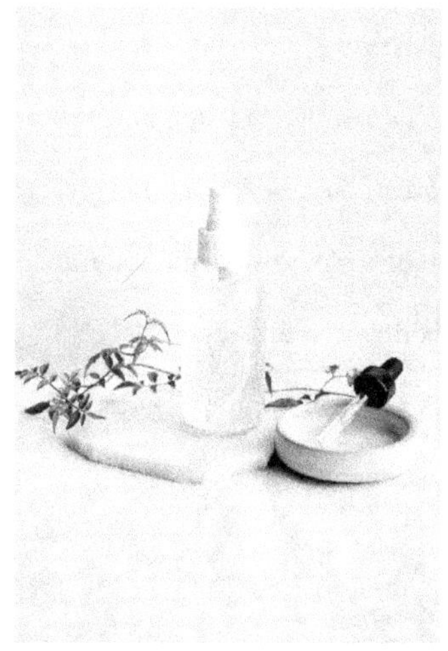

Directions:

Add ingredients into dark glass spray bottle and shake well before each use.

26. *Vanilla & Orange Natural Body Mist*

Ingredients:

- 20 drops of orange essential oil
- one teaspoon of vanilla extract
- half an ounce of vegetable glycerin
- half an ounce of witch hazel
- distilled water

Directions:

Shake all ingredients in a small glass spray bottle. Make sure to shake well before each use.

27. *Burst of Citrus Energy Body Mist*

Ingredients:

- half an ounce of witch hazel
- half an ounce of vegetable glycerin
- 20 drops of grapefruit essential oil
- six drops of lime essential oil
- six drops of lemon essential oil
- distilled water

Directions:

Mix all of your ingredients in a small glass spray bottle make sure to shake well before each use.

28. *Orange Blossom Body Mist*

Ingredients:

- 40 drops of orange essential oil
- one teaspoon of vegetable glycerin
- half an ounce of witch hazel
- distilled water

Directions:

Add ingredients into glass spray bottle and shake well. Shake before each use and when using it rub into skin.

29. *Patchouli Body Spray*

Ingredients:

- half a teaspoon of Tunisian Patchouli essential oil
- half an ounce of vegetable glycerin
- half an ounce of witch hazel
- distilled water

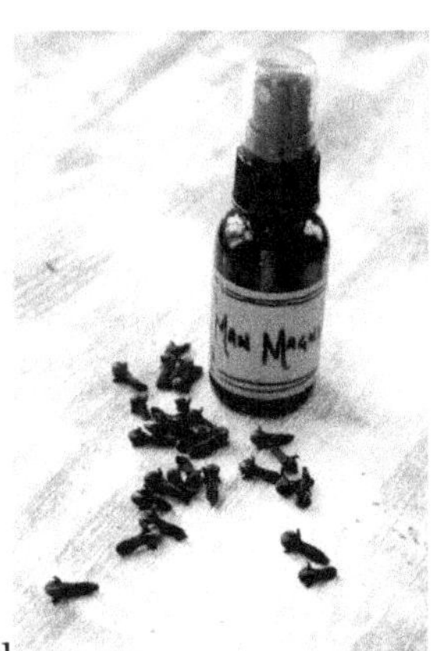

Directions:

Mix all ingredients in small glass spray bottle and shake well before each use.

30. *Vanilla Coffee Body Mist*

Ingredients:

- six coffee essential oil drops

- 20 vanilla oleoresin drops

- half an ounce of witch hazel

- distilled water

Directions:

Mix all ingredients in dark glass spray bottle. Shake well before each application.

31. *Sweet Orange & Vanilla Body Mist*

Ingredients:

- 20 vanilla oleoresin drops

- 20 sweet orange essential oil drops

- half an ounce of witch hazel

- distilled water

Directions:

Add all of your ingredients into small dark-glass spray bottle and make sure to shake before each use.

32. *Ylang-Ylang & Vanilla Body Mist*

Ingredients:

- 20 vanilla oleoresin drops

- four Ylang-Ylang essential oil drops

- half an ounce of witch hazel

- distilled water

Directions:

Add all of your ingredients into a dark-glass spray bottle make sure to shake well before each use.

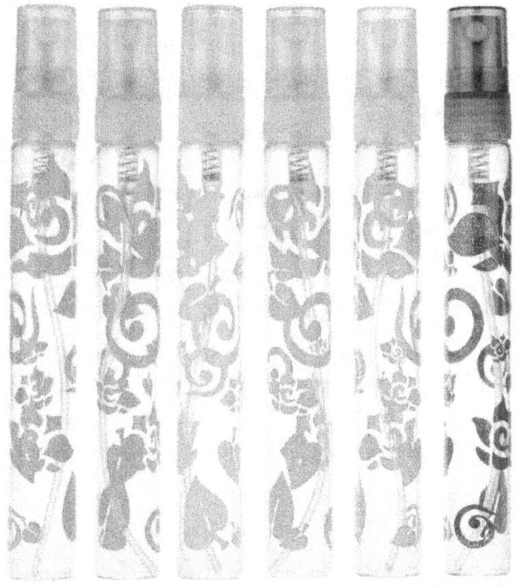

33. *Tea Tree Body Mist*

Ingredients:

- 25 drops of tea tree essential oil
- half an ounce of witch hazel
- distilled water

Directions:

Add your ingredients into a dark-glass spray bottle and shake well before each use.

34. *Marigold & Vanilla Body Mist*

Ingredients:

- 30 drops of marigold essential oil
- 20 drops of vanilla oleoresin
- half an ounce of witch hazel
- distilled water

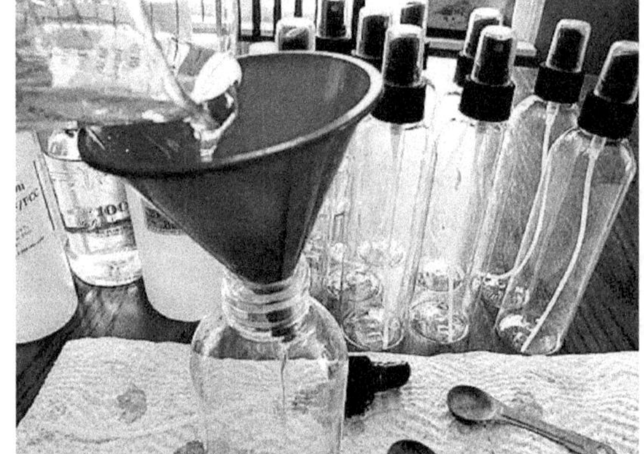

Directions:

Add all of your ingredients into dark-glass spray bottle shake well before each and every use. The scent of marigold in this spray will help to keep the pesky bugs at bay.

35. Raspberry & Lemon Body Mist

Ingredients:

- 25 raspberry essential oil drops

- 15 lemon essential oil drops

- half an ounce of witch hazel

- two tablespoons of vegetable glycerin

- distilled water

Directions:

Mix all ingredients in dark-glass spray bottle and shake before each and every use

.

Bonus Recipes for Homemade Perfumes!

36. Latenight Perfume

Ingredients:

- six tablespoons of witch hazel

- three tablespoons of Jojoba oil

- two and a half tablespoons of distilled water

- 10 drops of lavender essential oil

- 15 drops of clove essential oil

- 8 drops of cedarwood essential oil

Materials needed:

- coffee filter

- funnel

- two dark-glass spray bottles

Directions:

Clean the bottles out with some hot soapy water. You can also put them in your dishwasher to sterilize them. Add a lid to one of them and set it aside.

Add your carrier oil into one of the bottles. Add in essential oils. Add in witch hazel. Add lid to this bottle and shake well. Allow this bottle to rest for forty-eight hours to a couple of weeks.

The scent will be at its strongest at about six weeks. Check it weekly and once you get the scent you want add two tablespoons of distilled water and shake for a minute or so. Put the coffee filter into the funnel.

Transfer the liquid from the bottle it is in to a nice perfume bottle. Label it and store it in a cool and dark place.

37. *Lavender Citrus Homemade Perfume*

Ingredients:

- 15 drops of Bergamot essential oil
- 15 drops of lavender essential oil
- 12 drops of lemon essential oil
- 12 drops of sweet orange essential oil
- two teaspoons of beeswax
- two teaspoons of Jojoba oil

Directions:

Add your Jojoba oil and beeswax in a pan heat over medium heat until beeswax is melted. Remove from heat and add in essential oils mix well. Then add mix to small tin and allow to harden. Cover with lid.

38. Vanilla Lavender Perfume

Ingredients:

- 20 drops of lavender essential oil

- 15 drops of vanilla extract

- two vanilla beans

- once cup lavender flowers, dried

- two tablespoons of vegetable glycerin

- half a cup of witch hazel

Directions:

Using a sharp knife slice the vanilla beans open. Put the beans and the flowers in a large glass jar with a lid. Pour the witch hazel into the jar and secure the lid. Let this mix infuse for the next two weeks.

Strain with cheesecloth and discard lavender flowers and vanilla beans. Add the vegetable glycerin, vanilla extract and lavender essential oil to the reserved liquids and blend well. Put lid back onto jar and allow it to age for six weeks. Strain the perfume once again through a coffee filter then transfer it to a nice looking decorative spray bottle.

39. Sweet Citrus Sunshine Homemade Perfume

Ingredients:

- 10 drops of grapefruit essential oil

- 10 drops of sweet orange essential oil

- 10 drops of peppermint essential oil

- two tablespoons of witch hazel

- one tablespoon of Jojoba oil

- 10 drops of lavender oil

- distilled water

Directions:

Add jojoba oil to glass container then add in the witch hazel. Add in the essential oils and mix. Add in distilled water.

Transfer to a dark-glass container for up to six weeks. The longer you leave it to sit the stronger the scent will be. After you have reached the scent that you desire transfer into a nice attractive spray bottle.

40. Solid Organic Perfume

Ingredients:

- two tablespoons of beeswax

- 35 drops of lavender essential oil

- two tablespoons of olive oil

Directions:

In a double broiler add in your wax stir until melted then remove from heat. Add in the oils and pour into final container.

To use this wonderful solid perfume just wipe it on the interior of your wrist this will leave a wonderful clean scent that will last all day!

Conclusion

I hope that you will enjoy trying out my collection of deodorant, body sprays as well as the bonus homemade perfume recipes! Just think about how much better you are going to feel when you know that the non-toxic homemade organic deodorant you are using is not putting you at serious health risk such as developing breast cancer or Alzheimer's.

More and more people are looking to find the more natural approach to many aspects in life. We are becoming more aware and in tune with the harmful additives and chemicals that are filling many of the commercial products that we purchase on a day to day level. I wish you a happy and healthy journey towards living your life in a more natural and non-toxic way!

Thanks again for downloading my book, I really appreciate your support of my work. I would love to read your review of my book on Amazon. Happy making your new homemade deodorants, body sprays and perfumes! You smell great already!

FREE Bonus Reminder

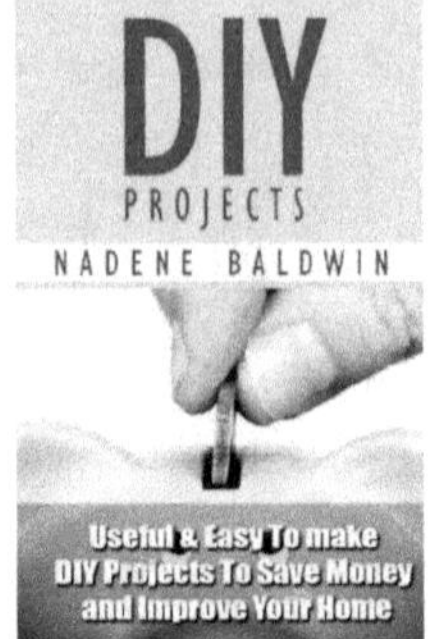

If you have not grabbed it yet, please go ahead and download your special bonus report *"DIY Projects. 13 Useful & Easy To Make DIY Projects To Save Money & Improve Your Home!"*
Simply Click the Button Below

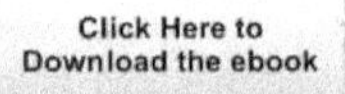

OR **Go to This Page**
http://diyhomecraft.com/free

BONUS #2: More Free & Discounted Books or Products
Do you want to receive more Free/Discounted Books or Products?
We have a mailing list where we send out our new Books or Products when they go free or with a discount on Amazon. Click on the link below to sign up for Free & Discount Book & Product Promotions.
=> Sign Up for Free & Discount Book & Product Promotions <=

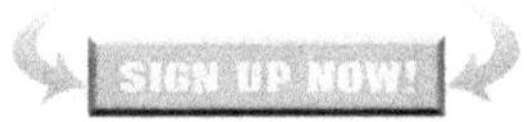

OR Go to this URL
http://zbit.ly/1WBb1Ek